Christmas Island Boat Disaster Response – Dr Fabian Schwarz

ASSESSMENT TASK 2: Written assignment

Aligned subject learning outcomes	<ul><li>Use sound public health science to advocate for the inclusion of ethical decision making within organisations</li><li>Articulate the significance of a multi-disciplinary approach to leadership and management during crises and disasters</li><li>Communicate to both professional and non-professional audiences the public health imperatives that mitigate the adverse effects of a crisis.</li></ul>
Aligned professional standards/ competencies	Justify population health activities by applying ethical principles including maleficence, beneficence, equity and justice.
	Location of peer-reviewed evidence based information (including Cochrane, Campbell etc)
	Analyse the management of a population health program during crisis in terms of strategic focus, organisational authority, leadership capacity, strategic partnerships, resource allocation, workforce capacity and mechanisms of accountability
Group or individual	Individual
Weighting	50%
Word Count	3000 words
Due date	29 May 2015

ASSESSMENT TASK 2: DESCRIPTION

Using a major **public health crisis or emergency** that has occurred since the year 2000, students must comprehensively critique the response to the event. Students should comment on the core topics introduced in TM5563.

a) Choose a major emergency or disaster that has occurred since the year 2000. Provide a BRIEF (no more than one paragraph) summary of the event.

b) Conduct a comprehensive literature review on the event. (Note: You may want to focus your search on the key management/leadership issues you want to address for the assignment). You must document a transparent search methodology, including search strategy, sources, date range searched, any limitations and results.

c) Using the literature identified, review and critique the response to the event. Students should comment on the core leadership / management topics introduced in TM5563. It may be useful to use clear subheadings for the issues you are examining.

d) Be sure to provide a reference list formatted in Vancouver style.

A) Christmas Island Disaster December 2010

50 international asylum seekers died in the coastal sea territory of Christmas Island on 15 December, 2010. The deceased were from a vessel identified by Australian authorities as Suspected Irregular Entry Vessel 221 ('SIEV 221'). The Western Australian State Coroner (1) reported that the event involved the largest peacetime loss of human life in a maritime incident in Australian waters during the last 115 years. SIEV 221 was dashed against rocks not far off the coast of Christmas Island; the exact cause is unclear, but a combination of engine-failure and rough seas are likely factors (1). Eye witnesses (2) reported seeing people, including women and children, drowning in the water.

SIEV 221
15 December 2010

We will reflect on this day with sadness.
The loss of each person's life diminishes our own because we are part of humankind.

AS YOU READ THIS PLEASE REMEMBER ALL ASYLUM SEEKERS WHO HAVE ATTEMPTED THIS TREACHEROUS JOURNEY

B) Literature review

1. Search strategy: Pubmed
   Search terms: Christmas Island Disaster response
   Limits: Last 5 years
   Results: 128 articles, none directly related to the Christmas Island Disaster described above.

2. Search strategy: JCU Library One Search
   Search terms: Christmas Island SIEV
   Limits: Scholarly & Peer Review, last 5 years
   Results: 27, none highly relevant.

3. Search strategy: JCU Library One Search
   Search terms: Christmas Island tragedy
   Limits: Scholarly & Peer Review, last 5 years
   Results: 1902, the top results composed primarily of opinion pieces.

4. Search strategy: Google
   Search terms: Christmas Island disaster response
   Limits: no limits set.
   Results: 590,000, choosing the first 5 pages to identify links of interest.

Identified key document: Inquiry into the incident of 15 Dec 2010. www.aph.gov.au/

Identified key documents: Coroners Report and Submission Inquiry

http://www.coronerscourt.wa.gov.au/_files/Christmas_Island_Findings.pdf

Identified collection of news articles:

http://www.safecom.org.au/siev221-lessons.htm

5. An additional reference search was conducted based on the articles and reports identified above, resulting in further key resources as follows:

   1. Emergency Management Review for the Indian Ocean Territories (3).
   2. The Christmas Island Emergency Management Plan Review (3).
   3. The internal Customs and Department of Defence review (18)
   4. The Parliamentary Committee of Inquiry (18)
   5. Coroner's Inquiry (8)

C) Core leadership and management topics in the Christmas Island SIEV disaster response

The boat disaster on Christmas Island led to the activation of an emergency management plan which was initially designed in January 2008 by the Emergency Management Committee. Optimal emergency management requires strong, coordinated and consultative relationships between government, non-government agencies and communities to allow for a fully integrated approach (3). Accounts of rescue efforts by frontline responders of the day confirmed that they had risked their own lives in order to save as many other lives as possible (1-3). Whilst critiques (5-7) applauded the mariners for their heroic rescue efforts, they nonetheless raised a number of essential questions regarding internal Border Protection Command (BPC) communication, policy, decision-making, and response times.

This paper is a review of key leadership issues during the response phase of the Christmas Island crisis. Several internal and external reviews relating to the emergency management response and arrangements on Christmas Island (3, 8, 18) have been consulted to assess the quality of the core leadership and management of the disaster response. Topics that will be examined in relation to the disaster include: leadership, managing media and communication, psychosocial aspects, ethical challenges, standards of care, management challenges in mass fatality events, legal issues and standards, and legal and professional obligations of responders. Although the principal components of prevention and preparedness are paramount for disaster management (1), these will not be covered further because they are beyond the scope of this paper. Some references to the recovery phase efforts, such as search and recovery and morgue operations, will be made in order to assess these aspects of the crisis leadership during the Christmas Island boat disaster.

1. Leadership during crisis

An assessment of leadership during the boat disaster is an important measure to take in order to better appreciate the effectiveness of the emergency response. The Christmas Island Emergency Plan (3) stipulates that the Territory Controller (TC) is the key person responsible for overall management of an emergency response. The Australian Federal Police usually designates a senior officer for this purpose (9). The TC advises the Island Administrator and the Emergency Management Committee (EMC) during an emergency and can request Australian Government assistance (3). The EMC contains representatives from local organisations and has to rely on local resources during a disaster due to the island's remote location and isolation. It is important to note that Christmas Island has a strong sense of community, and volunteers staff a large number of the emergency services such as ambulance, SES, fire service and VMRS (10) which ultimately receive their instruction from the TC. The leadership displayed by the TC during the event was described by the duty doctor (3) as having done an 'excellent job' at coordinating the incident and patient off-loading sites. A further reflection by the same doctor (4) went on to suggest that the disaster management plan 'worked very well' as the staff were able to cope with the magnitude of the event, and only a few survivors of the mass casualty population needed to be evacuated to the mainland. Despite this, the Joint Select Committee on the Christmas Island Tragedy (3) mentioned that the EMC was not 'functioning as effectively as it could be' and that it was in need of 'strong leadership' so that it could be recognised by the community as having a meaningful role. The committee also felt that the EMC was relying too heavily 'on committed key individuals' rather than a system which provides structured roles and training programs for emergency relief help. It is important to note that key appointments in the EMC were based on two year terms (AFP TC and Island Administrator) which posed an increased risk for lack of continuity and local knowledge because of staff changeover. Also, contact lists were found to be out of date (3). The Coroner's report (8) suggested that there was some challenge with raising the initial alarm across the responsible agencies implying that some deficit in situational awareness possibly delayed the initial response to the disaster. Critics (3,5) emphasised that there was not enough information provided to the patrol boat(s) early on in the disaster, and that aircraft and mainland resources were not fully coordinated by the TC. Federal political leaders were also criticised for a lack of situational awareness in the handling of the aftermath of the boat disaster (11).

Although there was only limited information available about leadership visibility, availability, effective risk communication and self-control, it is clear that the conduct of the TC effectively corresponded with the Christmas Island Emergency Management Plan. Suggestions about how to improve the effectiveness of leadership involved altering the emergency management plan and personal setup in order to minimise gaps in communication; this would have increased the reliability and the continuity of the emergency response system.

2. Managing media and communication during crisis

Crisis leadership requires optimal communication with all stakeholders, which ultimately includes the media. Therefore, it is necessary to review the system in place, and how it is utilised. The Christmas Island communication system relies on 'spectrum radio, mobile phones, landlines and satellite internet services' (3). This system is considered to be adequate for emergency management purposes for Christmas Island (3). However, even before the Christmas Island disaster, the unreliability of this communication model in poor weather conditions had been identified by critics as a problematic issue (10). Nonetheless, on the day of the boat disaster, communication between on-island agencies and the mainland was 'extensive' and 'co-operative' (3). No deficiencies were identified with the actual on-island response to the incident as a result of the communication system. Also, senior staff met on the day of the incident in Canberra and liaised with the Border Protection Taskforce (BPT) (3). However, the Christmas Island Emergency Management Committee (EMC) (3) identified a lack of communication resources and procedure knowledge (for example availability and use of radios), which made it challenging to communicate during the emergency response. EMC members were also not fully aware of the routine 'DIAC-suspect-boat-arrivals procedures', revealing a lack of consensual and conceptual communication and understanding (3). Furthermore, airport management was not consulted about incoming aircrafts, causing a deficit in communication and oversight; this was due to a lack of consultation between on-island and mainland agencies, who had not fully entrusted the local community and Territory Controller (TC) with the management of the emergency recovery. Since the TC was not fully aware of all the movements of aircraft and mainland resources, there may have been a 'duplication of effort' or 'wasted resources' (3). As expected, the incident gained significant media coverage with ten journalists flying to the site of the crisis within hours, providing an opportunity for interaction with the media on-site (2, 3, 11). However, the Minister for Home Affairs took over communication with the press as the disaster unfolded and provided frequent press statements off-site (3).

It appears that the media was managed well and that communication protocols were followed as far as they had been known or established. Criticism was focused mainly on the lack of on-site communication equipment, lack of recognition of local leadership, and difficulties with off-site resource coordination.

3. Psychosocial aspect of crisis management

It is recognised that those involved in a crisis can experience significant levels of distress (10, 13); this requires consideration when discussing crisis management, because all those exposed to a crisis can be affected. Crisis management demands an awareness of particular stress factors and calls for local knowledge and cultural considerations (10, 13). Provision of information and appropriate communication can assist those in distress, as these meet immediate needs and create confidence (12). In addition, appropriate and effective crisis management decreases stress levels, and allows for optimal psychosocial aftercare (12).

Appropriate psychosocial responses to disaster are demonstrated in the Christmas Island incident via the different agencies on the island who dealt with the event internally (3). Unfortunately, there is only limited information available about the immediate on-site mental health first aid during the emergency response. However, it is clear that survivors, aid providers and the Christmas Island community were strongly affected by the tragedy. The community memorial ceremony held shortly after the crisis clearly indicated the impact of the tragedy on many people beyond the frontline and survivors thanked the Christmas Island residents for their support. (13). The Commonwealth provided funding for ongoing counselling services for helpers and Christmas Island community members in the recovery phase. However, there are several notable media reports (15) that criticize the Australian government's means of addressing the psychosocial care of the victims in the disaster aftermath. The psychological impact on the survivors is difficult to quantify, and ongoing detention of the survivors is a grave concern. The practice of long-term mandatory detention adds to the mental health burden on the island since it is noted by health professionals (14) that events such as these have significant mental health implications. From this, even though there can be significant mental health complications from such disasters on victims, there can also be an impact on first responders. For example, Dr Sarah Giles (4) was the duty doctor on Christmas Island at the time, and she referred to the tragedy as a life-changing event for herself. Dr Sarah Giles (4) reported ongoing guilt and a sense of loss, but also found a new sense of purpose for her own life. This kind of response exemplifies the psychosocial impact a crisis situation can have on those exposed to it and how good crisis leadership can assist with recovery from distress.

4. Ethical challenges and crisis management

Crisis situations pose ethical challenges and dilemmas relating to the standard of care, leadership and decision making, legal issues and the appropriate handling of mass casualties. This section will examine the events on Christmas Island from an ethical and legal perspective using the aforementioned key ideas.

a) Standards of care during disaster

The standard of care during the Christmas Island boat disaster was as effective as it could have been based on the resources and help available (3-4, 8). Brian Lacy (3), the Island Administrator at the time, described the rescue response as 'heroic', mentioning the bravery of both naval personnel and community members. The coroner (8), also commended the prompt and efficient actions of the Navy (with Lieutenant Commander Livingstone aboard HMAS Pirie, and Andrew Stammers, Master of the ACV Triton). However, Leading Seaman Boatswain Mate Jonathan West (8) drew attention to the fact that decisions about standards of care were still very challenging to make, citing that after collecting ten survivors it was necessary for him to return to HMAS Pirie for offloading. Leading Seaman West was required to make a decision about turning around to save his own life and the lives of those on-board, but also expressed the difficulties of seeing survivors, whom he had to leave behind, in the water trying to climb on-board.

As well, duty doctor Giles (4) raised the challenging question of whether the accident could have been prevented. Dr. Giles hypothesised that if healthcare professionals had refused to work on Christmas Island due to the questionable ethics of detention facilities, then the facilities would not have existed, and refugees would not have attempted to reach the Island at all. Instead, this arrangement would have forced the Australian government to undertake on-shore processing; therefore, facilities on Christmas Island would not have been in use. This, in turn, would have possibly reduced the extent of the boat tragedy due to the arrival of fewer boats. Dr. Giles also added that she felt complicit in the loss of human life, describing herself as being a 'cog in a machine that ultimately lured 48 people to their deaths'. Despite this, in summary, Dr. Giles reported that the standard of care during the emergency response was not compromised; she explained that the emergency management plan was instrumental in saving dozens of lives.

b) Leadership and management during emerging crises

A key challenge for a leader during an emerging crisis is effective risk and crisis communication (16-17). Risk communication is a 'dynamic and interactive process involving exchanges between different groups of key players and audiences (including the public)' (16). Risk communication is based on ongoing projections and calculations of the potential for future harm. Conversely, crisis communication is a 'spontaneous and reactive process, often occurring in unexpected emergency situations' (17). Crisis communication deals with an existing or emerging event and is based on current knowledge about the event (or lack thereof) (17). However, both terms are often used interchangeable in the literature (16-17).

Community involvement is crucial to providing effective relief during an emergency, and is integral to appropriate risk communication. During the emergency response of the Christmas Island boat disaster, it was imperative that a two-way exchange of information between the Territory Controller (TC) and the frontline rescuers was maintained. Due to the fact that many of the Christmas Island rescuers were local volunteers, it is clear that the wider community should be treated as a relevant audience for the purpose of crisis communication during emergency relief. For example, one volunteer rescuers (18) emphasised how inextricable the local community is from risk and crisis communication when he expressed that residents on Christmas Island should be entitled to the

TC's information about refugee boats; this is due to the fact that the residents of Christmas Island are the first responders during a boat disaster, and therefore feel a deep emotional impact and responsibility towards asylum seekers. The idea of community involvement was also supported by a report released by the Joint Select Committee on the Christmas Island Tragedy (18) when they acknowledged the enormous risk taken by rescuers to save lives. Furthermore, one of the rescue commanders explained that it is of utmost importance for any individual to provide aid where possible, and that he was confident that his team members were capable in making sound judgements that balanced rescue efforts and personal safety. Good crisis leadership is therefore enhanced by relevant risk and crisis communication with well-trained team members and requires a mutual understanding (16-18). This was evident on Christmas Island because crisis communication was concise and gave the individuals involved the responsibility to act based on their perception of the risks involved. Accordingly, emergency training for rescue volunteers was flagged as a key requirement by the Joint Select Committee on the Christmas Island Tragedy (18). Lastly, the harbourmaster and Territory Controller (TC) (18) in charge on the day deemed the launching of boats from the island to be an 'unacceptable risk due to dangerous weather conditions' and therefore prevented Christmas Island residents from doing so. This decision was based on a risk assessment and reflects good leadership during an emerging crisis. Additionally, the decision also ensured the safety of all volunteer rescuers involved. Overall, the leadership during the Christmas Island boat tragedy demonstrated appropriate and effective risk and crisis communication without any significant identifiable deficits.

c) Leadership and management during mass fatality events

Two important issues during mass fatality events are 'search and recovery' and 'morgue operations' which can make the crisis management response extra challenging as seen on Christmas Island. The search and recovery efforts during the Christmas Island incident were severely limited due to the harsh weather and a lack of suitable search and rescue vessels (18). The local morgue had the capacity to hold six bodies; thus, the island administration organised a chiller container to serve as a temporary morgue. Body bags were scarce and therefore supply was organised through the Western Australian Department of Health (18). As well, the Department of Health provided forensic specialists and equipment in order to aid with the relief efforts. The Royal Flying Doctor Service (RFDS) also provided staff and resources for retrieval purposes (18). This emphasises that the Christmas Island leadership team had to source and rely on interagency help to mount an appropriate crisis response. A crisis response for a mass fatality event can be divided into three phases:

- *Phase 1: responders arrive at scene, incident command structures setup*
- *Phase 2: disaster plan activated, responders in designated roles*
- *Phase 3: resolution, removal of bodies, family support, recovery*

Each phase will be fully investigated below in relation to the Christmas Island response.

Phase 1 started when Christmas Island residents spotted a boat (SIEV 221), which had lost engine power and was drifting towards the cliffs just off Rocky Point where it would later sink. The residents responded immediately by throwing life jackets into the water (3). Mr. Murray (18), one of the locals present on the day, recounted his feelings of helplessness and hopelessness, vividly describing seeing a woman trying to save her baby; he also described the event as occurring in 'slow motion' and in his close proximity. Along with accounts like this, the review committee also heard that none of the refugees would have escaped with their lives had it not been for the life jackets thrown from the rocks by the Christmas Island residents (18).

Subsequent to the sighting of the boat, government agencies including the Australian Federal Police (AFP), the Australian Customs and Border Protection and the Australian Defence Force (ADF) were alerted and the situation was escalated to a 'Safety of Life at Sea [SOLAS] situation' (18). Lieutenant Commander

Mitchell Livingstone (19) reported that he and his crew had prepared for a boarding of the SIEV based on tentative information regarding the presence of a suspected vessel in Flying Fish Cove. However 20 minutes later, the event became a distress call and finally a 'mass SOLAS situation'. Livingstone went on to explain that 'worst-case scenarios' are always kept 'in mind' and therefore the speeds of responses are always optimal and change very little (19). In summary it can be said that the response to phase 1 was appropriate based on available information.

Phase 2 began with the activation of the Emergency Management Plan (EMP) by the Territory Controller (TC) at 06:20am. The process was reported as 'smooth and effective' (3). Relevant government offices in Perth and Canberra also received information in the morning hours of the incident (3). Christmas Islands' health service mobilised staff and equipment and set up triage facilities at the offloading boat ramp. As well, St. John's ambulance volunteers transported survivors in need of treatment to facilities atop Phosphate Hill. From there, retrieval and transport to facilities on the mainland could be organised (3). The Emergency Management Committee (EMC) staff were also involved in the rescue efforts and held meetings every three hours. Service delivery arrangements were tested and proved successful, allowing for resources to be brought to the island from the mainland (3).

The island administrator and the TC managed to oversee the incident site and the boat ramp offloading site at Ethel beach. HMAS Pirie and ACT Triton arrived at the scene at 07:05am and 07:14am respectively - these were deemed to be efficient response times (18). The Joint Select Committee on the Christmas Island Tragedy (18) noted that the total rescue effort was well coordinated, and did not lead to the loss of additional lives despite the significant risk posed to rescuers. This point of view was echoed by a report (18) provided by the Customs Supervisor which stated that the ship and crew were operating at their 'absolute limit', meaning few changes to procedures and equipment could be made to further improve their response. The report went on to detail that boundaries were truly tested since the 'sea state' of the day reached a level of '7 to 8', whilst the ship had an operational capacity reaching only '3 to 4'; however, it was suggested that this was a necessity in order to save lives (20).

Overall, the leadership and response to phase 2 were timely and in line with the Emergency Management Plan. Criticism was limited to minor points around procedures and equipment which did not impact on the overall response.

Phase 3 commenced after the initial emergency response was completed and no further survivors were found in the water. The Joint Select Committee on the Christmas Island Tragedy (18) detailed that, under the auspices of the Australian Federal Police customs officers at Christmas Island assisted with the offloading of survivors and decreased at Ethel Beach from 11:00am until around 5:00pm. Additional resources arrived, and the dead bodies were removed over the subsequent days. At this point, the Australian Maritime Safety Authority (AMSA) took over the search and rescue responsibility and completed the mission on 17 December, 2010 (18).

Support for victims, their families, and those involved in the rescue mission was also made available. Local volunteers played an important role in the recovery operation. Dr. Julie Graham (10, 18) provided some insight into the nature of the assistance offered by local drivers, saying that they were 'asked and readily agreed and went out to help'. Counselling services for all volunteer drivers were provided immediately after the incident and proceeded on a long-term basis under the control of the Indian Ocean Territories Health Service (IOTHS) (21). The review committee praised the IOTHS for its outstanding efforts in identifying and providing psychological support to individuals in need after the incident. Additional team members were deployed to the island to help with the ongoing counselling services (18). The first funerals were organised in February of 2011 which was criticised by some of the victims' family members (22). There were also delays in funeral arrangements due to the complexities of identifying the deceased (22). A community memorial service was held on 5 March, 2011 and was attended by key personnel from all major agencies involved in the relief effort. This was described by some as an 'intrinsic part of the healing process for the community' (18). An entire chapter is dedicated to the after-care of the survivors in the report handed down by the Joint Select Committee on the Christmas Island Tragedy. The review committee (18) said that they were mindful of the 'deep trauma experienced by the survivors' and said that they believed that 'appropriate care and support had been provided'. It was also recommended by the committee (18) that the Department of Immigration and Citizenship (DIAC) 'continue to monitor the wellbeing of survivors' and that 'support services should be provided for as long as necessary'.

In summary, the crisis response throughout all phases was appropriate and timely. The response also demonstrated sound decision-making skills when it came to search and rescue efforts, morgue operations and aftercare for the local population and survivors. However, there are challenges and concerns about the ongoing care for survivors while in detention facilities.

d) Legal issues during crisis management

In general, a legal framework is required to allow rescuers to provide an appropriate crisis response (23-25, 27). The Christmas Island boat disaster can be viewed as a crime scene with the crisis response informed by just legal standards and professionals acting within their legal obligations. (23-25, 27)

Christmas Island legal status quo

The current legal framework on Christmas Island was established in 1992 by the Territories Law Reform Act. The Christmas Island Disaster management plan was not supported by legislation (23). In actual fact, the Territory of Christmas Island is directly under Commonwealth legislation, making the Attorney General the minister responsible for emergency management matters (3).

Disaster as crime scene

The coronial inquest into the Christmas Island SIEV 221 tragedy on 15 December, 2010 lasted between May 2011 and February 2012, ending when Western Australian Coroner handed down his findings about the disaster. The coroner had made 'an open finding' as to the cause of death for the refugees (24). The report (8) suggested rescue workers, both professionals and volunteers, did what they could with the resources they had available. A criminal investigation based on human trafficking laws was undertaken, and three Indonesian men were charged in January, 2011 (25).

Legal standards during disaster

From an international perspective, disasters are a human rights issue and victims of a disaster have the right to life and the right to adequate shelter and medical treatment (26). From an Australian perspective, legislation around disasters is generally implemented at the state and territory level with very little applicable national legislation (27). The boat disaster on Christmas Island was handled well according to the legal standards discussed in the Australian Emergency Handbook for Disaster Health (27). Accurate documentation of the incident was recorded which is essential to both ensure continuity of patient care and allow for the preparation and prevention of future disasters. An awareness of appropriate occupational health and safety issues prevented injury and harm to health care workers. Overall, the standard of care provided during the boat disaster was as effective as possible based on the available resources and conditions (19, 21).

Legal and professional obligations of first responders

International and Australian law oblige every vessel at sea to do what is possible to render assistance to vessels in distress (28). First responders, including doctors, are covered by Good Samaritan protection laws which state that a 'Good Samaritan' is any person who in 'good faith and without expectation of payment or reward' provides assistance to an injured person, or person at risk of injury (29). Medical practitioners are professionally and ethically obligated to act as Good Samaritans (29). Good Samaritan provisions also apply in emergency situations. In the event that a doctor does render aid, he or she may be covered by Good Samaritan protection against civil litigation (30). Literature on the subject is unclear about the legal and professional obligations for non-medical staff in emergency situations; however, should a doctor refuse to render assistance where a duty of care is supposed, there is potential for a negligence case to be successfully leveled against their name. It is important to note that in these cases, it is not possible to know with absolute certainty how the courts will judge such matters (30). Overall, the Christmas Island crisis response was within the framework of the Commonwealth legislation for emergency management and professional and legal obligations and standards were followed accordingly by first responders. There has been no criticism around the legal matter pertaining to the Christmas Island crisis response and leadership.

Conclusion

The response to the Christmas Island disaster was determined to be as effective as possible considering the adverse weather conditions, remote location and resource availability. The Emergency Management Plan (EMP) worked well and leadership during the event was strong and effective. The Territory Controller (TC) demonstrated good risk and crisis communication during the disaster. However, despite this there are some valid critiques of the response; as such, lessons have been learnt from the incident and addressed. For example it resulted in the need for employing a community Emergency Management Officer to assist with continuity of operations knowledge requisition and risk communication.

The review committee pointed out that the events of the day were well-documented and directed particular attention to the bravery of Christmas Island residents and personnel aboard HMAS Pirie and HMAS Triton. An internal review carried out by Customs and Border Protection detailed the events that occurred on the morning of 15 December, 2010. The review examined the effectiveness of internal policies and found that all standard procedures were followed by the agency. The review also made eight recommendations in response to the 'lessons learned from the event', five of which were readily implemented with the remaining three pending completion at the time of the review's submission. The review committee concluded that all relevant people and agencies acted in accordance with established policies. The committee believed that all applicable responses were undertaken, and expressed satisfaction with interagency cooperation and communication that was coordinated during the crisis. Lastly, the committee did not identify anything throughout the course of its inquiry relating to the rescue efforts mounted that was suggestive of inadequacy or of particularly poor quality. Legal and professionals standards were adhered to which facilitated an appropriate search and recovery response and mass casualty management.

5. References

1. Vogl A. Coroner says Christmas Island tragedy was 'foreseeable'. Alternative Law Journal 2012;37(2):139. Available from:
http://www.coronerscourt.wa.gov.au/_files/Christmas_Island_Findings.pdf

2. News report. Dozens feared dead in asylum wreck horror. ABC News. 15 Dec 2010. Available from:
http://www.abc.net.au/news/2010-12-15/dozens-feared-dead-in-asylum-wreck-horror/2375126

3. Australian Government. Department of Regional Australia, Regional Development and Local Government. Submission to the joint select committee inquiry into the incident of 15 December 2010. Joint Select Committee on the Christmas Island Tragedy. 27 April 2011. Available from:
http://www.aph.gov.au/DocumentStore.ashx?id=f5f319be-fa3d-44d1-b7c7-65c9be2c3790

4. Giles S. If you're not part of the solution. Narrative Inquiry in Bioethics. 2013;3(2): E11-E13. Available from
http://search.proquest.com/docview/1469903860?accountid=16285

5. Kevin T. Reluctant rescuers: an exploration of the Australian border protection system's safety record in detecting and intercepting asylum-seeker boats, 1998-2011 / Tony Kevin T. Kevin Manuka,

A.C.T 2012. ISBN 9780987319005. Available from: http://reluctantrescuers.com/Reluctant-Rescuers.pdf

6. Kevin T. Questions surround latest asylum seeker boat disaster [online].Eureka Street. Dec 2011;21(24): 28-30. Available from: http://search.informit.com.au.elibrary.jcu.edu.au/documentSummary;dn=795734965510914;res=IELAPA ISSN: 1036-1758. [cited 16 May 15].

7. Kevin T. Personal Reflections on the Christmas Island Tragedy [online]. Eureka Street. Dec 2010;20(24): 13-15. Available from: http://search.informit.com.au.elibrary.jcu.edu.au/documentSummary;dn=635403934489899;res=IELAPA ISSN: 1036-1758. [cited 16 May 15].

8. Coroner's Court of Western Australia. Record of Investigation: Christmas Island Tragedy. 23 February 2012. Available from: http://www.coronerscourt.wa.gov.au/_files/Christmas_Island_Findings.pdf

9. Australian Government. Attorney-General's Department. Australian Emergency Management: Christmas Island arrangements. Available from: http://www.em.gov.au/Emergencymanagement/Preparingforemergencies/Plansandarrangements/Pages/ChristmasIslandArrangements.aspx)

10. Schwarz F. Personal knowledge from working at Christmas Island Hospital in 2013.

11. SafeCom. The SIEV-221 drama: lessons from a disaster. 2011. Available from: http://www.safecom.org.au/siev221-lessons.htm

12. Schedlich C. Psychosocial Crisis Management in CBRN incidents. Council of Europe, Strasbourg. 2014. Available from: http://www.coe.int/t/dg4/majorhazards/activites/2014/ClaudiaSchedlich_PSCMinCBRN.pdf

13. Briskman L, Fiske L, Dimasi M. The impact of Australian asylum seeker policy on Christmas Islanders (2001-2011). Shima: The International Journal of Research into Island Cultures. 6(2):99-115. Available from: http://www.shimajournal.org/issues/v6n2/j.%20Briskman%20et%20al%20Shima%20v6n2%2099-115.pdf

14. Procter, NG. Mental Health Implications of the Christmas Island Boat Crash Tragedy. Contemporary Nurse: A Journal for the Australian Nursing Profession. Feb 2011; 37(2): 111-11.

15. Cowie T. Is Christmas Island prepared for boat tragedy? 16 December 2010. Crikey. Available from: http://www.crikey.com.au/2010/12/16/is-christmas-island-adequately-prepared-for-boat-tragedy/?wpmp_switcher=mobile

16. Covello VT, Sandman PM. Risk communication: evolution and revolution. In: Wolbarst A, editor. Solutions to an environment in peril. Baltimore: John Hopkins University Press; 2001. p.164-78.

17. Infanti J, Sixsmith J, Barry M M, et al. A literature review on effective risk communication for the prevention and control of

communicable diseases in Europe. Stockholm: ECDC; 2013. Available from: http://ecdc.europa.eu/en/publications/Publications/risk-communication-literary-review-jan-2013.pdf

18. Parliament of Australia. Joint Select Committee on the Christmas Island Tragedy. 2011. Available from: http://www.aph.gov.au/Parliamentary_Business/Committees/Joint/Former_Committees/christmasisland/christmas_island/report/c03

19. Lieutenant Commander Mitchell Livingstone. Commanding Officer, HMAS Pririe, Navy, ADF. Proof Committee Hansard. 2011:5.

20. Mr Mathew Saunders. Customs Supervisor, Customs, Proof Committee Hansard. 2011:5.

21. Dr Julie Graham. Director, Indian Ocean Territory Health Service. 2010.

22. ABC News. Christmas Island funerals anger relatives. Retrieved 13 May 2015. http://www.abc.net.au/news/2011-02-15/christmas-island-funerals-anger-relatives/1942970)

23. Australian Government. Attorney-General's Department. Australian Emergency Management: Christmas Island arrangements. Available from: http://www.em.gov.au/Emergencymanagement/Preparingforemergencies/Plansandarrangements/Pages/ChristmasIslandArrangements.aspx

24. Australian Government. Department of Infrastructure. Annual Report. 2011. Available from: https://www.infrastructure.gov.au/department/annual_report/2011_2012/regional/part03/chap08/chap08_external_scrutiny.html

25. BBC News. Three charged over Christmas Island shipwreck. Retrieved 13 May 2015. http://www.bbc.com/news/world-asia-pacific-1227293926

26. Eburn M. Law's contribution to emergency and disaster management. ANU. 2012. Available from: http://www.bushfirecrc.com/sites/default/files/managed/resource/northumbria_7_december_2012.pdf

27. Australian Emergency Handbook 1. Chapter 16 Legal issues, documentation and occupational health. Available from: www.em.gov.au

28. Kaye S. Maritime search and rescue as everyone's responsibility. Australian Journal of Maritime and Ocean Affairs. 2011;3(4): 136-137. Available from: http://search.proquest.com/docview/1010049407?accountid=16285

29. Bird S. Good Samaritans. Australian Family Physician. 2008;37(7): 570-1.

30. Bird S. Duty of care or a matter of conduct. Australian Family Physician. 2013;42(10):746-748.